Table of Contents

What Is the Optavia Diet?

The Optavia Diet is the brainchild of the man behind the multimillion-dollar company Medifast– Dr. William Vitale. Now carrying the brand Optavia since 2017, the goal of this diet is to encourage healthy and sustainable weight loss among its clientele. While there are many types of diet regimen that are available in the market, the Optavia Diet is ranked in the top 30 Best Diets in the United States.

Under this diet regimen, dieters are required to follow a weight plan that includes five feelings a day and one lean green meal daily. However, there are also other regimens of the Optavia Diet if the five fuelings a day is too much for you. And since this is a commercial diet, you have access to Optavia coaches and become part of a community that will encourage you to succeed in your weight loss journey. Moreover, this diet is also designed for people who want to transition from their old habits to healthier ones. Basically, this diet regimen is not only for people who want to lose weight but also for people who suffer from diabetes, people suffering from gout, nursing moms, seniors as well as teens.

The Optavia Diet has been subjected to various studies to prove its efficacy in weight loss. Different studies were published in various journals indicating that those who follow this program are able to see significant changes in as little as 8 weeks and that people can achieve their long-term health goals with the Optavia Diet.

The Benefits of The Optavia Diet

The Optavia Diet, similar to other weight loss programs, promises people a high success rate. However, unlike other programs, this particular diet regimen is not only easy to follow but it is also great for those who have long-term health goals. Thus, below are the benefits of following this diet regimen.

- **Structured Eating Plan:** The Optavia Diet has a structured eating plan thus making it one of the most no-brainer diets there is. Everything is spelled out for you so there is no need for you to figure out if you are following the diet correctly. Since it is very easy to follow, it is perfect for people who are always busy or do not have a knack for cooking their food.

- **Great for People Practicing Portion Control:** One of the most challenging parts of dieting is learning how to do portion control and sticking by it. The Optavia Diet comes with the Fueling phase that helps keep your meals in check so there is no need for you to eat unnecessarily.

- **Practice Long-Term Relationship with Food:** The guidance of the community following the Optavia Diet can help improve a positive long-term relationship with food. Over time, you become aware of the types of foods that you are allowed to eat and gain an appreciation of the healthy options that you have.

- **Does Not Need an Accountability Partner:** While some diets encourage you to have a diet buddy, the Optavia Diet is perfect for people who do not have accountability partners. The thing is that people are connected to a community of dieters that can provide the support needed while going through the phases of this diet.

- **Better Overall Health:** This particular diet regimen is known to help improve overall wellness. Aside from weight loss, various studies have also noted that the Optavia Diet can help people maintain stable blood pressure and blood sugar levels due to the limited sodium intake that the food contains. In fact, the Optavia provides less than 2,300 milligrams of Sodium daily.

A Deeper Look into The Optavia Diet

The Optavia Diet encourages people to limit the number of calories that they should take daily. Under this program, dieters are encouraged to consume between 800 and 1000 calories daily. For this to be possible, dieters are encouraged to opt for healthier food items as well as meal replacements. But unlike other types of commercial diet regimens, the Optavia Diet comes in different variations. There are currently three variations of the Optavia Diet plan that one can choose from according to one's needs.

- **5&1 Optavia Diet Plan:** This is the most common version of the Optavia Diet and it involves eating five prepackaged meals from the Optimal Health Fuelings and one home-made balanced meal.
- **4&2&1 Octavia Diet Plan:** This diet plan is designed for people who want to have flexibility while following this regimen. Under this program, dieters are encouraged to eat more calories and have more flexible food choices. This means that they can consume 4 prepackaged Optimal Health Fuelings food, three home-cooked meals from the Lean and Green, and one snack daily.
- **5&2&2 Optavia Diet Plan:** This diet plan is perfect for individuals who prefer to have a flexible meal plan in order to achieve a healthy weight. It is recommended for a wide variety of people. Under this diet regimen, dieters are required to eat 5 fuelings, 2 lean and green meals, and 2 healthy snacks.
- **3&3 Optavia Diet Plan:** This particular Diet plan is created for people who have moderate weight problems and merely want to maintain a healthy body. Under this diet plan, dieters are encouraged to consume 3 prepackaged Optimal Health Fuelings and three home-cooked meals.

- **Optavia for Nursing Mothers:** This diet regimen is designed for nursing mothers with babies of at least two months old. Aside from supporting breastfeeding mothers, it also encourages gradual weight loss.
- **Optavia for Diabetes:** This Optavia Diet plan is designed for people who have Type 1 and Type 2 diabetes. The meal plans are designed so that dieters consume more green and lean meals depending on their needs and condition.
- **Optavia for Gout:** This diet regimen incorporates a balance of foods that are low in purines and moderate in protein.
- **Optavia for Seniors (65 years and older):** Designed for seniors, this Optavia Diet plan has some variations following the components of Fuelings depending on the needs and activities of the senior dieters.
- **Optavia for Teen Boys and Optavia for Teen Girls (13-18 years old):** Designed for active teens, the Optavia for Teens Boys and Optavia for Teens Girls provide the right nutrition to growing teens.

Regardless of which type of Optavia Diet plan you choose, it is important that you talk with a coach to help you determine which plan is right for you based on your individual goals. This is to ensure that you get the most out of the plan that you have chosen.

How to Start This Diet

The Optavia Diet is comprised of different phases. A certified coach will educate you on the steps that you need to undertake if you want to follow this regimen. But for the sake of those who are new to this diet, below are some of the things that you need to know especially when you are still starting with this diet regimen.

Initial Steps

During this phase, people are encouraged to consume 800 to 1,000 calories to help you shed off at least 12 pounds within the next 12 weeks. For instance, if you are following the 5&1 Optavia Diet Plan, then you need to eat 1 meal every 2 or 3 hours and include a 30-minute moderate workout most days of your week. You need to consume not more than 100 grams of carbohydrates daily during this phase.

Further, consuming the Lean and Green meals are highly encouraged. It involves eating 5 to 7 ounces of cooked lean proteins and three servings of non-starchy vegetables, and two servings of healthy fats. This phase also encourages the dieter to include 1 optional snack per day such as ½ cup sugar-free gelatin,3 celery sticks, and 12 ounces nuts. Aside from these things, below are other things that you need to remember when following this phase:

- Make sure that the portion size recommendations are for cooked weight and not the raw weight of your ingredients
- Opt for meals that are baked, grilled, broiled, or poached. Avoid frying foods as this will increase your calorie intake.
- Eat at least two servings of fish rich in Omega-3 fatty acids. These include fishes like tuna, salmon, trout, mackerel, herring, and other cold-water fishes.
- Choose meatless alternatives like tofu and tempeh.
- Follow the program even when you are dining out. Keep in mind that drinking alcohol is discouraged when following this plan.

Maintenance Phase

As soon as you have achieved your desired weight, the next phase is the transition stage. It is a 6-week stage that involves increasing your calorie intake to 1,550 per day. This is also the phase when you are allowed to add more varieties into your meal such as whole grains, low-fat dairy, and fruits.

After six weeks, you can now move into the 3&3 Optavia Diet plan, so you are required to eat three Lean and Green meals and 3 Fueling foods.

What CAN I Eat and NOT Eat?

There are so many foods that you can eat while following the Optavia Diet. However, you must know these foods by heart. This is especially true if you are just new to this diet and you have to strictly follow the 5&1 Optavia Diet Plan. Thus, this section is dedicated to the types of foods that you are allowed and not allowed to eat while following this diet regimen.

Foods That Are Allowed

There are several categories of foods that can be eaten under this diet regimen. This section will break down the Lean and Green foods that you can eat while following this diet regime.

The Lean Foods

Leanest Foods - These foods are considered to be the leanest as it has only up to 4 grams of total fat. Moreover, dieters should eat a 7-ounce cooked portion of these foods. Consume these foods with 1 healthy fat serving.

- **Fish:** Flounder, cod, haddock, grouper, Mahi, tilapia, tuna (yellowfin fresh or canned), and wild catfish.
- **Shellfish:** Scallops, lobster, crabs, shrimp
- **Game meat:** Elk, deer, buffalo
- **Ground turkey or other meat:** Should be 98% lean
- **Meatless alternatives:** 14 egg whites, 2 cups egg substitute, 5 ounces seitan, 1 ½ cups 1% cottage cheese, and 12 ounces non-fat 0% Greek yogurt

Leaner Foods - These foods contain 5 to 9 grams of total fat. Consume these foods with 1 healthy fat serving. Make sure to consume only 6 ounces of a cooked portion of these foods daily:

Fish: Halibut, trout, and swordfish

- **Chicken:** White meat such as breasts as long as the skin is removed
- **Turkey:** Ground turkey as long as it is 95% to 97% lean.
- **Meatless options:** 2 whole eggs plus 4 egg whites, 2 whole eggs plus one cup egg substitute, 1 ½ cups 2% cottage cheese, and 12 ounces low fat 2% plain Greek yogurt

Lean Foods - These are foods that contain 10g to 20g total fat. When consuming these foods, there should be no serving of healthy fat. These include the following:

- **Fish:** Tuna (bluefin steak), salmon, herring, farmed catfish, and mackerel
- **Lean beef:** Ground, steak, and roast
- **Lamb:** All cuts
- **Pork:** Pork chops, pork tenderloin, and all parts. Make sure to remove the skin
- **Ground turkey and other meats:** 85% to 94% lean
- **Chicken:** Any dark meat
- **Meatless options:** 15 ounces extra-firm tofu, 3 whole eggs (up to two times per week), 4 ounces reduced-fat skim cheese, 8 ounces part-skim ricotta cheese, and 5 ounces tempeh

Healthy Fat Servings - Healthy fat servings are allowed under this diet. They should contain 5 grams of fat and less than grams of carbohydrates. Regardless of what type of Optavia Diet plan you follow, make sure that you add between 0 and 2 healthy fat servings daily. Below are the different healthy fat servings that you can eat:

- 1 teaspoon oil (any kind of oil)
- 1 tablespoon low carbohydrate salad dressing
- 2 tablespoons reduced-fat salad dressing
- 5 to 10 black or green olives
- 1 ½ ounce avocado
- 1/3-ounce plain nuts including peanuts, almonds, pistachios
- 1 tablespoon plain seeds such as chia, sesame, flax, and pumpkin seeds
- ½ tablespoon regular butter, mayonnaise, and margarine

The Green Foods

This section will discuss the green servings that you still need to consume while following the Optavia Diet Plan. These include all kinds of vegetables that have been categorized from lower, moderate, and high in terms of carbohydrate content. One serving of vegetables should be at ½ cup unless otherwise specified.

Lower Carbohydrate - These are vegetables that contain low amounts of carbohydrates. If you are following the 5&1 Optavia Diet plan, then these vegetables are good for you.

- **A cup of green leafy vegetables** such as collard greens (raw), lettuce (green leaf, iceberg, butterhead, and romaine), spinach (raw), mustard greens, spring mix, bok choy (raw), and watercress.
- **½ cup of vegetables** including cucumbers, celery, radishes, white mushroom, sprouts (mung bean, alfalfa), arugula, turnip greens, escarole, nopales, Swiss chard (raw), jalapeno, and bok choy (cooked).

Moderate Carbohydrate - These are vegetables that contain moderate amounts of carbohydrates. Below are the types of vegetables that can be consumed in moderation:

- **½ cup of any of the following vegetables** such as asparagus, cauliflower, fennel bulb, eggplant, portabella mushrooms, kale, cooked spinach, summer squash (zucchini and scallop).

Higher Carbohydrates - Foods that are under this category contain a high amount of starch. Make sure to consume limited amounts of these vegetables.

- **½ cup of the following vegetables** like chayote squash, red cabbage, broccoli, cooked collard and mustard greens, green or wax beans, kohlrabi, kabocha squash, cooked leeks, any peppers, okra, raw scallion, summer squash such as straightneck and crookneck, tomatoes, spaghetti squash, turnips, jicama, cooked Swiss chard, and hearts of palm.

Foods That Are Not Allowed

There are many types of foods that are not allowed for the Optavia Diet Plan. These foods either contain high amounts of fats or carbohydrates that can contribute to weight gain. Below are the types of foods that are not allowed under this particular diet:

- Fried foods
- Alcohol
- Milk
- Cheese
- Fruit juice
- Soda and other sweetened beverages
- Refined grains such as pasta, white rice, and white bread

How Easy Is This Diet to Follow?

When embarking on any new diet regimen, you may experience some difficulties along the way. Below are the reasons why this diet regimen is considered as the easiest to follow among all commercial diet regimens.

- **Eating out can be challenging but still possible:** If you love eating out, you can download Optavia's dining out guide. The guide comes with tips on how to navigate buffets, order beverages, and choose condiments. Aside from following the guide, you can also ask the chef to make substitutions for the ingredients used in cooking your food. For instance, you can ask the chef to serve no more than 7 ounces of steak and serve it with steamed broccoli instead of baked potatoes.

- **Opt for lean and green foods that have high fullness index:** Eat foods that contain high protein and fiber content as they can keep you full for longer periods. In fact, many nutrition experts highlight the importance of satiety when it comes to weight loss.

- **You have access to knowledgeable coaches:** If you follow the Optavia Diet plan, you have access to knowledgeable coaches and become a part of a community that will give you access to support calls and community events. You also have a standby nutrition support team that can answer your questions.

Optavia Diet Plans FAQs

You may have some questions about the Optavia Diet Plan. Below are some of the common FAQs that people ask about this diet regimen.

Which program is right for me?

Optavia offers a wide variety of programs that are designed to improve health and well-being. Choosing the right one is easy as these diet plans are designed for different individuals and their needs. However, if you are still not sure about which diet plan to follow, you can always get in touch with an Optavia coach to learn about the many options that you have.

Is it okay for me to skip fuelings?

Fuelings is very important as it is specifically formulated with the right balance of macronutrients (carbohydrates, fats, and protein). Proper fueling can help promote an efficient fat-burning state so that people lose fat without losing their energy. If you skip fueling, you might miss out on these important nutrients including your daily dose of vitamins and minerals. Now, if you accidentally skip your fuelings within 24 hours, it is crucial to double up so that you don't miss the nutrition provided by your fuelings.

Which plan is best for my level of fitness?

Exercise can lead to lifelong transformation. This is the reason why specific Optavia Diet plan is designed for people who have different activity levels. Active adults who engage in 45 minutes of light to moderate exercise can benefit from the 5&1 Plan. Always talk with your coach on which plan is great for your age and activity level.

Can I rearrange my fuelings especially if I work on long days or night duty?

Yes. You can rearrange the timing of your fuelings depending on your schedule. What is important is that you consume your fuelings and lean and green meals within 24 hours. So, whether you work at night or on regular hours, make sure that you eat your meals every 2 or 3 hours throughout the time that you are awake.

How often should I eat my meals?

The Optavia Diet plan teaches you the habit of eating healthy. You are encouraged to eat six small meals daily. As mentioned earlier, you are encouraged to eat every two to three hours from your waking time. Thus, start your day with fuelings and eat your lean and green meals in between your fuelings. It is recommended that you eat your first meal within an hour of waking to ensure optimal blood sugar. This is also a good strategy for hunger control.

Lean and Green Recipes

Chicken Stir Fry

Serves: 2
Cooking Time: 1 minutes

Ingredients:
- ½ cup chicken broth, low sodium
- 12 ounces skinless chicken breasts, cut into strips
- 1 cup red bell pepper, seeded and chopped
- 8 ounces (1 cup) broccoli, cut into florets
- 1 teaspoon crushed red pepper

Directions:
1. Place a small amount of chicken broth in a saucepan. Heat over medium flame and stir in the chicken. Water sauté the chicken for at least 5 minutes while stirring constantly.
2. Place the rest of the ingredients and stir.
3. Cover the pan with lid and cook for another 5 minutes.

Nutrition Information:
Calories per serving: 137; Protein: 15g; Carbs: 15.4g; Fat: 1.2g Sugar: 0.6g

Optavia Tomato Basil Soup

Serves: 2
Cooking Time: 10 minutes

Ingredients:
- 1 cup tomatoes, chopped
- ½ cup water
- 1 cup basil leaves
- 1 tablespoon low-sodium and low-fat cheese, shredded

Directions:
1. Place the tomatoes in a saucepan. Pour water. Close the lid.
2. Turn the heat to medium and allow the tomatoes to boil.
3. Using a handheld blender, puree the tomatoes while still in a pan.
4. Add in the basil leaves and allow to cook for another 2 minutes.
5. Scoop in bowls and serve with ½ tablespoon each shredded cheese.

Nutrition Information:
Calories per serving: 137; Protein: 1.7g; Carbs: 3g; Fat: 0.9g Sugar: 0.9g

Lean and Green Cauliflower Salad

Serves: 2
Cooking Time: 3 minutes

Ingredients:
- 1 cup cauliflower florets
- ¼ cup apple cider vinegar
- 1 tablespoon Tuscan seasoning

Directions:
1. Add all ingredients into a bowl and toss to combine.
2. Allow to rest in the fridge for at least 30 minutes before serving.

Nutrition Information:
Calories per serving: 41; Protein: 1.3g; Carbs: 8.7g; Fat: 0.1g Sugar: 2g

Lean and Green Garlic Chicken with Zoodles

Serves: 5
Cooking Time: 10 minutes

Ingredients:
- 1 ½ pounds boneless and skinless chicken breasts, cut into bite-sized pieces
- 6 slices sun-dried tomatoes
- 1 teaspoon chopped garlic
- 1 cup low fat plain Greek yogurt
- ½ cup chicken broth, low sodium
- ½ teaspoon garlic powder
- ½ teaspoon Italian seasoning
- 1 cup spinach, chopped
- 1 ½ cup zucchini, cut into thin noodles

Directions:
1. Place 2 tablespoons water in a pan and heat over low-medium flame. Water sauté the chicken for 3 minutes while stirring constantly until the sides are slightly golden.
2. Stir in the tomatoes and garlic and stir for another 3 minutes. Add in the yogurt, chicken broth, garlic powder, and Italian seasoning. Cover with lid and allow to simmer for at least 7 minutes.
3. Stir in the spinach last. Cook for another 2 minutes.
4. Place the zucchini noodles in a deep dish and pour over the chicken. Toss the noodles to coat with the sauce.
5. Serve immediately.

Nutrition Information:
Calories per serving: 205; Protein: 33.3g; Carbs: 6g; Fat: 2g Sugar: 1.2g

Lean and Green "Macaroni"

Serves: 4
Cooking Time: 10 minutes

Ingredients:
- 2 tablespoons yellow onion, diced
- 5 ounces 95-97% lean ground beef
- 2 tablespoons light thousand island dressing
- 1/8 teaspoon apple cider vinegar
- 1/8 teaspoon onion powder
- 3 cups Romaine lettuce, shredded
- 2 tablespoons low-fat cheddar cheese, shredded
- 1-ounce dill pickle slices
- 1 teaspoon sesame seeds

Directions:
1. Put 3 tablespoons of water in a pan and heat over medium-low flame. Water sauté the onions for 30 seconds before adding the beef. Sauté the beef for 4 minutes while stirring constantly.
2. Add in the thousand island dressing, apple cider vinegar, and onion powder. Close the lid and keep on cooking for 5 minutes. Remove the lid and allow to simmer until the sauce thickens. Turn off the heat and allow the beef to rest and cool.
3. In a bowl, place the lettuce at the bottom and pour in the beef. Layer with cheddar cheese, and pickles. Sprinkle with sesame on top.

Nutrition Information:
Calories per serving:119; Protein: 10.8g; Carbs: 4.4g; Fat: 2.1g Sugar: 2.5g

Lean and Green Broccoli Taco

Serves: 4
Cooking Time: 15 minutes

Ingredients:
- 4 ounces 95-97% lean ground beef
- ¼ cup roma tomatoes, chopped
- ¼ teaspoon garlic powder
- ¼ teaspoon onion powder
- 1 ¼ cup broccoli, cut into bite-sized pieces
- A pinch of red pepper flakes
- 1 ounce low-sodium cheddar cheese, shredded

Directions:
1. Place 3 tablespoons of water in a pan and heat over medium flame. Water sauté the beef and tomatoes for 5 minutes until the tomatoes are wilted. Add in the garlic and onion powder and stir for another 3 minutes.
2. Add the broccoli and close the lid. Cook for another 5 minutes.
3. Garnish with red pepper flakes and cheddar cheese on top.

Nutrition Information:
Calories per serving:97; Protein:9.9 g; Carbs: 2.6g; Fat: 1.7g Sugar:0.9 g

Lean and Green Crunchy Chicken Tacos

Serves: 4
Cooking Time: 10 minutes

Ingredients:
- ½ cup low sodium chicken stock
- 2 chicken breasts, minced
- 1 red onion, chopped
- 1 clove of garlic, minced
- 3 plum tomatoes, chopped
- 1 teaspoon cumin powder
- 1 teaspoon cinnamon powder
- 1 teaspoon ground coriander
- 1 red onion, chopped
- ½ red chili, chopped
- 1 tablespoon lime juice
- Meat from 1 ripe avocado
- 1 cucumber, sliced into thick rounds

Directions:
1. Place a tablespoon of chicken stock in a pan and heat over medium flame. Water sauté the chicken, onion, garlic, and tomatoes for 4 minutes or until the tomatoes have wilted.
2. Season with cumin, cinnamon, and coriander. Reduce the heat to low and cook for another 5 minutes. Set aside and allow to cool.
3. In a bowl, mix together the onion, chili, lime juice, and mashed avocado. This is the salsa.
4. Scoop the salsa and top on sliced cucumber. Top with cooked chicken.

Nutrition Information:
Calories per serving: 313; Protein: 31.8g; Carbs: 14.9 g; Fat: 3.8g Sugar: 5g

Optavia-Approved Vegetarian Zucchini Lasagna

Serves: 6
Cooking Time: 10 minutes

Ingredients:

- 1 ¼ pounds zucchini, sliced into lasagna
- ¼ cup chopped fresh spinach
- 1 ½ cup sugar-free and low-sodium marinara sauce
- 2/3 cup mozzarella cheese, shredded
- 1 cup part-skim ricotta cheese
- Fresh basil for garnish

Directions:

1. Preheat the oven to 375^0F for 5 minutes.
2. Place the zucchini slices in a dish and layer with spinach, marinara sauce, mozzarella, and ricotta cheese. Repeat the process until several layers are formed.
3. Top with basil.
4. Place in the oven and bake for 10 minutes.

Nutrition Information:

Calories per serving: 128; Protein: 12.2g; Carbs: 10.7g; Fat: 2.6g Sugar: 2.1g

Cauliflower with Kale Pesto

Serves: 6
Cooking Time: 2 minutes

Ingredients:
- 3 cups cauliflower, cut into florets
- 3 cups raw kale, stems removed
- 2 cups fresh basil
- 2 tablespoons extra virgin olive oil
- 3 tablespoons lemon juice
- 3 cloves of garlic
- ¼ teaspoon salt

Directions:
1. Put enough water in a pot and bring to a boil over medium flame. Blanch the cauliflower for 2 minutes. Drain then place in a bowl of ice-cold water for 5 minutes. Drain again.
2. In a blender, add the rest of the ingredients. Pulse until smooth.
3. Pour over the pesto over the cooked cauliflower.

Nutrition Information:
Calories per serving: 41; Protein: 1.8g; Carbs: 5g; Fat: 5.3g; Sugar: 1.4g

Lean and Green Chicken Chili

Serves: 6
Cooking Time: 45 minutes

Ingredients:
- 1-pound boneless skinless chicken breast, chopped
- 1 teaspoon ground cumin
- 1 cup chopped poblano pepper
- ½ cup chopped onion
- 1 clove of garlic, minced
- 2 cups low-sodium chicken broth
- 1 cup rehydrated pinto beans
- 1 cup chopped tomatoes
- 2 tablespoons minced cilantro

Directions:
1. Place all ingredients except the cilantro in a pressure cooker.
2. Close the lid and set the vent to the sealing position.
3. Cook on high for 45 minutes until the beans are soft.
4. Garnish with cilantro before serving.

Nutrition Information:
Calories per serving: 229; Protein: 26.1g; Carbs: 23.9g; Fat: 2g Sugar: 2.2g

Avocado, Citrus, And Shrimp Salad

Serves: 4
Cooking Time: 4 minutes

Ingredients:
- 1 head green leaf lettuce
- 1 avocado
- ½ pound wild-caught shrimp
- 2 tablespoons olive oil
- Juice of 1 lemon

Directions:
1. Place the lettuce in a bowl and top with mashed avocado meat.
2. Clean the shrimps by deveining and removing the head.
3. Heat oil in a skillet over medium low heat and heat the oil. Cook the shrimps for 2 minutes on each side.
4. Place the shrimps on top of mashed avocado and drizzle with lemon juice.

Nutrition Information:
Calories per serving: 359; Protein: 10.6g; Carbs: 50.1g; Fat: 7.5g Sugar: 2.8g

Lean and Green Broccoli Alfredo

Serves: 5
Cooking Time: 2 minutes

Ingredients:
- 2 heads of broccoli, cut into florets
- 2 tablespoons lemon juice, freshly squeezed
- ½ cup cashew, soaked for 2 hours in water then drained
- 2 tablespoons white miso, low sodium
- 2 teaspoon Dijon mustard
- Freshly cracked black pepper

Directions:
1. Boil water in a pot over medium flame. Blanch the broccoli for 2 minutes then place in a bowl of iced water. Drain.
2. In a food processor, place the remaining ingredients and pulse until smooth.
3. Pour the alfredo sauce over the broccoli. Toss to coat with the sauce.

Nutrition Information:
Calories per serving: 359; Protein: 10.6g; Carbs: 50.2 g; Fat: 8.4g Sugar: 2.4g

Lean and Green Steak Machine

Serves: 3
Cooking Time:10 minutes

Ingredients:
- 1/2 teaspoon extra virgin olive oil
- 2 ounces Sirloin steak, 98% lean
- Salt and pepper to taste
- 1 zucchini, cut into long thin strips
- 1 onion, chopped
- 6 ounces asparagus, blanched
- 4 ounces peas, blanched

Directions:
1. Heat olive oil in a skillet. Season the steak with salt and pepper to taste.
2. Place in the skillet and sear the steak for 5 minutes on each side. Allow to rest for five minutes before slicing into strips.
3. Place the remaining ingredients in a bowl and season with salt and pepper to taste
4. Top with steak strips then toss to combine all ingredients.

Nutrition Information:
Calories per serving:174; Protein: 4.2g; Carbs: 10.3g; Fat: 4.1g Sugar: 2.1g

Garlic Shrimp Zucchini Noodles

Serves: 5
Cooking Time: 4 minutes

Ingredients:
- 16 ounces uncooked shrimps, shelled and deveined
- 1 tablespoon olive oil
- 1 cup cherry tomatoes, cut in half
- 8 cups zucchini strips
- 2 tablespoons minced garlic
- 1 teaspoon dried oregano
- ½ teaspoon chili powder
- ½ teaspoon salt

Directions:
1. Brush the shrimps with olive oil. Place on a skillet and cook for 2 minutes on all sides or until pink. Set aside.
2. Place the rest of the ingredients in a bowl and add the shrimps. Season with salt then toss to coat the ingredients.

Nutrition Information:
Calories per serving: 142; Protein: 19.7g; Carbs: 6.3g; Fat: 4.2g Sugar: 3.8g

Lean and Green Crockpot Chili

Serves: 8
Cooking Time: 45 minutes

Ingredients:
- 1-pound boneless skinless chicken breasts, cut into strips
- ½ cup chopped onion
- 2 teaspoons ground cumin
- 1 teaspoon minced garlic
- ½ teaspoon chili powder
- Salt and pepper to taste
- 1 ½ cups water
- 1 can green enchilada sauce
- ½ cup dried beans, soaked overnight

Directions:
1. Place all ingredients in a pot.
2. Mix all ingredients until combined.
3. Close the lid and turn on the heat to medium.
4. Bring to a boil and allow to simmer for 45 minutes or until the beans are cooked.
5. Serve with chopped cilantro on top.

Nutrition Information:
Calories per serving: 84; Protein: 13.4g; Carbs: 3.6 g; Fat: 1.7g Sugar: 0.8g

Garlic Herb Mashed Cauliflower

Serves: 5
Cooking Time: 10 minutes

Ingredients:
- 1 head cauliflower, cut into florets
- 3 cloves of garlic, minced
- ¼ cup plain Greek yogurt
- 2 teaspoons chopped thyme
- 2 teaspoons chopped rosemary
- Salt and pepper to taste

Directions:
1. Put enough water in a pot and bring to a boil.
2. Place the florets in a large pot and cook for 10 minutes or until soft. Drain the cauliflower.
3. Place the drained cauliflower in a blender together with the remaining ingredients.
4. Pulse until smooth.

Nutrition Information:
Calories per serving: 25; Protein: 2.2g; Carbs: 4.5g; Fat: 0.2g Sugar: 0.7g

Spaghetti Squash with Buffalo Sauce

Serves: 6
Cooking Time: 15 minutes

Ingredients:
- 1 pound skinless and boneless chicken breasts, cut into strips
- ½ cup chicken stock, low sodium
- ½ cup red hot sauce
- ½ teaspoon garlic powder
- 2 ½ pounds spaghetti squash, halved and seeded
- 8 ounces cream cheese, low sodium

Directions:
1. Place the chicken breasts in a deep saucepan. Stir in the stock, hot sauce, and garlic powder. Stir to combine all ingredients.
2. Place a rack or a steamer on top of the pot and place the spaghetti squash.
3. Cover with lid.
4. Bring to a boil and allow to simmer for 10 to 15 minutes.
5. Once cooked, take the spaghetti squash out of the steamer, and allow to rest. Using a fork, scrape the spaghetti squash and place on a plate.
6. Mix in the cream cheese into the chicken sauce.
7. Pour the sauce over the spaghetti squash.

Nutrition Information:
Calories per serving: 273; Protein: 21.6g; Carbs: 16.1g; Fat: 3.2g Sugar: 3.1g

Skinny Shrimp Scampi with Zucchini Noodles

Serves: 4
Cooking Time:4 minutes

Ingredients:
- 1 teaspoon olive oil
- 1 tablespoon minced garlic
- 1-pound jumbo shrimps, shelled and deveined
- ¼ teaspoon crushed red pepper flakes
- 5 tablespoons water
- 2 tablespoons lemon juice, freshly squeezed
- 2 medium zucchinis, spiralized into noodles then blanched
- Chopped parsley for garnish

Directions:
1. Heat oil in a saucepan over medium flame.
2. Sauté the garlic for 30 seconds before adding in the shrimps. Stir for another 30 seconds before putting in the red pepper flakes, water, and lemon juice.
3. Allow to cook for 3 minutes while stirring constantly. Season with salt and pepper if desired.
4. Place the blanched zucchini on a plate and pour on top the shrimps.
5. Garnish with parsley if desired.

Nutrition Information:
Calories per serving:136; Protein: 23.9g; Carbs: 2.6 g; Fat: 1.8g Sugar: 0.5g

Lean and Green Chicken and Green Beans

Serves: 5
Cooking Time: 9 minutes

Ingredients:
- 1 teaspoon extra virgin olive oil
- 2 teaspoons minced garlic
- 1-pound boneless chicken breasts, cut into strips
- 2 ½ cups green beans, trimmed and cut into 1-inch pieces
- ¼ cup water
- Salt and pepper to taste

Directions:
1. Place oil in a saucepan and heat over medium flame. Sauté the garlic for 30 seconds until fragrant.
2. Add in the chicken breasts and continue to cook for another 3 minutes while stirring constantly.
3. Add in the green beans and water. Scrape the bottom of the pan to remove the browning.
4. Season with salt and pepper to taste.
5. Close the lid and allow to simmer for 6 minutes.

Nutrition Information:
Calories per serving: 198; Protein: 21.3g; Carbs: 4.5 g; Fat: 3.5g Sugar: 2.1g

Shrimp and Cauliflower Grits

Serves: 4
Cooking Time: 15 minutes

Ingredients:
- 1 large head cauliflower, cut into small florets
- 1 cup 1% milk
- 1 tablespoon unsalted butter
- Salt and pepper to taste
- 1 ¼ pounds deveined shrimps
- A pinch of cayenne pepper
- Chopped parsley for garnish

Directions:
1. Place the cauliflower in a food processor and pulse until the florets break into finer pieces resembling grits or grains of rice. Place the cauliflower grits into a saucepan and add the milk, ½ of the butter, salt, and pepper. Allow to simmer over medium heat for 10 minutes while stirring constantly. Remove from the heat and allow to rest.
2. Season the shrimps with salt and pepper. Brush a clean pan with the remaining of the butter and cook the shrimps for 2 minutes on each side over low-medium flame. Set aside.
3. Assemble the dish by placing cauliflower mash on a plate. Serve with shrimps on top and garnish with cayenne pepper and parsley.

Nutrition Information:
Calories per serving:227; Protein: 33.3g; Carbs: 9.3 g; Fat: 2.5g Sugar: 4.1g

Healthy Fish Patties

Serves: 3
Cooking Time: 6 minutes

Ingredients:
- 10 ounces flounder fillet, chopped finely
- 1/3 cup celery stalk, chopped finely
- 1/3 cup red pepper, chopped finely
- 1 tablespoon fresh dill, chopped finely
- 2 teaspoons Dijon mustard
- 2 eggs, slightly beaten
- Salt and pepper to taste

Directions:
1. Place all ingredients in a bowl. Mix until well-incorporated.
2. Form small patties with your hands and place on a baking sheet. Allow patties to rest in the fridge for at least 30 minutes.
3. Brush pan with extra virgin olive oil and allow to heat over medium flame.
4. Place individual patties into the pan and cook for 3 minutes on each side.
5. Serve immediately.

Nutrition Information:
Calories per serving: 380; Protein: 28.7g; Carbs: 13g; Fat: 5.4g Sugar: 0.02g

One Pot Taco Zucchini Noodles

Serves: 6
Cooking Time: 20 minutes

Ingredients:
- 1 tablespoon olive oil
- 1-pound lean ground turkey
- 1 clove garlic, minced
- ½ small onion, chopped
- 1 tablespoon chili powder
- ¼ teaspoon garlic powder
- ¼ teaspoon onion powder
- ¼ teaspoon dried oregano
- 1 ½ teaspoon ground cumin
- ¼ cup water
- ¼ cup diced tomatoes
- 2 large zucchinis, spiralized
- ½ cup shredded cheddar cheese

Directions:
1. Place oil in a pot and heat over medium flame.
2. Sauté the turkey for 2 minutes before adding the garlic and onions. Stir for another minute.
3. Season with chili powder, garlic powder, onion powder, oregano, and ground cumin. Sauté for another minute before adding the water and tomatoes.
4. Close the lid and allow to simmer for 7 minutes.
5. Add in the zucchini and cheese and allow to cook for 3 more minutes.

Nutrition Information:
Calories per serving: 145; Protein: 15g; Carbs: 8.5g; Fat:2.1 g Sugar: 0.5g

Green Big Mac Salad

Serves: 6
Cooking Time: 7 minutes

Ingredients:
- 1 pound 98% lean ground beef
- A pinch of salt
- ¼ teaspoon black pepper
- 8 ounces Romaine lettuce, torn
- 1 cup cherry tomatoes, halved
- ½ cup pickles, diced
- ¼ cup cheddar cheese, shredded

Directions:
1. Season the beef with salt and pepper.
2. Heat a non-stick pan and sauté the beef white stirring constantly for 7 minutes. Set aside and allow to slightly cool.
3. Place the lettuce, tomatoes, pickles, and cheese. Sprinkle the cooked beef on top.
4. Toss to mix all ingredients.

Nutrition Information:
Calories per serving: 186; Protein: 21g; Carbs: 8.7g; Fat: 3.1g Sugar: 0.8g

Green Monster Veggie Burger

Serves: 6
Cooking Time: 10 minutes

Ingredients:
- 1 cup broccoli florets
- 1 cup green peas
- 1 cup baby spinach
- ¼ cup chickpea flour
- 1 teaspoon paprika powder
- 1 teaspoon cumin powder
- Salt according to taste

Directions:
1. Place all ingredients in a food processor and pulse until smooth.
2. Using your hands, form patties using the mixture and place on a baking sheet.
3. Brush extra virgin olive oil on a non-stick pan and cook the burger for 5 minutes over medium-low flame on both sides or until all sides are golden.

Nutrition Information:
Calories per serving: 40; Protein: 2.6g; Carbs: 6.3g; Fat: 0.4g Sugar: 1g

Broccoli and Tomato Salad

Serves: 3
Cooking Time: 2 minutes

Ingredients:
- 1 head broccoli, cut into florets then blanched
- ¼ cup tomatoes, diced
- Salt and pepper to taste
- Chopped parsley for garnish

Directions:
1. Place all ingredients in a bowl.
2. Toss to coat all ingredients.
3. Serve.

Nutrition Information:
Calories per serving: 52; Protein: 1.1g; Carbs: 3.2g; Fat: 0.1g Sugar: 0.2g

Turkey Stuffed Zucchini Boats

Serves: 8
Cooking Time: 20 minutes

Ingredients:
- 4 medium zucchinis
- 2 tablespoons extra virgin olive oil
- 1-pound lean ground turkey
- 3 cloves of garlic, minced
- ½ onion, chopped
- ½ green pepper, seeded and chopped
- ½ cup skimmed mozzarella cheese, shredded

Directions:
1. Prepare the zucchini by slicing them in half lengthwise. Scoop the meat out. Chopped the scooped-up zucchini meat and set aside.
2. Heat oil in a saucepan over medium flame. Stir in the turkey and garlic and sauté for 5 minutes.
3. Stir in the onions halfway while the turkey is cooking. Add in the green pepper and zucchini meat. Cook for another 3 minutes. Set aside to cool completely.
4. Once cooled, stir in the mozzarella cheese.
5. Fill the hollowed-out zucchini with the meat mixture.
6. Place in a 360^0F preheated oven and bake for 10 minutes.

Nutrition Information:
Calories per serving: 115; Protein: 13.2g; Carbs: 6.3g; Fat: 1.4g Sugar: 0.5g

Mexican Cauliflower Rice Skillet

Serves: 6
Cooking Time: 11 minutes

Ingredients:
- 1 pound 98% lean ground beef
- ¼ medium onion, diced
- ½ teaspoon red pepper, diced
- 1 tablespoon chili powder
- ¼ teaspoon garlic powder
- ¼ teaspoon onion powder
- ¼ teaspoon dried oregano
- 1 ½ teaspoon ground cumin
- 1 cup diced tomatoes
- 12 ounces cauliflower rice or grits
- ½ cup water
- 1 ½ cup low sodium cheddar cheese

Directions:
1. Place the beef on a non-stick pan and sauté together with the onion, red pepper, chili powder, garlic powder, onion powder, dried oregano, and cumin. Stir constantly for 3 minutes until lightly golden.
2. Stir in the tomatoes and cook for another 3 minutes.
3. Add in the cauliflower grits and water.
4. Close the lid and cook for another 5 minutes.
5. Turn off the heat and stir in the cheddar cheese on top.

Nutrition Information:
Calories per serving: 352; Protein: 29g; Carbs: 7g; Fat: 5g Sugar: 3g

Lean and Green Buddha Bowl

Serves: 6
Cooking Time: 10 minutes

Ingredients:
- 2 pounds boneless and skinless chicken breast
- 2 tablespoons lemon juice, freshly squeezed
- Salt and pepper to taste
- 1-pound Brussels sprouts, trimmed and halved
- 3 cloves of garlic, minced
- ¾ cup plain Greek yogurt
- 1 teaspoon stone-ground mustard
- ¼ cup balsamic vinegar
- 2 cups cooked quinoa
- 1 cup chopped red apple, cored, and chopped
- ¼ cup pepitas
- 1 avocado, sliced
- 1 ½ cup arugula
- 1 tablespoon fresh basil

Directions:
1. Place chicken and lemon juice in a bowl. Season with salt and pepper to taste. Allow to marinate in the fridge for at least 30 minutes.
2. Fire up the grill to 375°F and cook the chicken for 6 minutes on each side. Add in the Brussels sprouts and cook for 3 minutes on each side. Set the chicken and Brussels sprouts aside.
3. In a bowl, mix together the garlic, yogurt, mustard, and vinegar. Season with salt to taste. Set aside.
4. On a bowl, place the quinoa and top with apple, pepitas, avocado, and arugula. Top with grilled chicken and Brussels sprouts.
5. Drizzle with the sauce and garnish with basil.

Nutrition Information:
Calories per serving: 411; Protein: 44.2g; Carbs: 40.4g; Fat: 4g Sugar: 3g

Garlic-Parmesan Tilapia

Serves: 4
Cooking Time: 10 minutes

Ingredients:
- 4 tilapia fillets
- 2 tablespoons extra-virgin olive oil
- Juice from 1 lemon
- 1 teaspoon garlic powder
- ¼ cup grated Parmesan cheese
- Salt and pepper to taste
- A bowl of fresh arugula

Directions:
1. Preheat the grill to 300^0F for 5 minutes.
2. Place tilapia on a baking sheet lined with foil.
3. In a bowl, mix the olive oil, lemon juice, and garlic powder.
4. Brush the fish with the oil mixture on all sides.
5. Sprinkle with parmesan cheese, salt, and pepper on all sides.
6. Place fish in the grill and cook for 5 minutes on each side.
7. Serve on top of arugula leaves.

Nutrition Information:
Calories per serving: 149; Protein: 25.8g; Carbs: 13.2g; Fat: 2.1g Sugar: 0.9g

Raw Zucchini Noodles with Pesto

Serves: 4
Cooking Time: 2 minutes

Ingredients:
- 2 medium zucchinis, spiralized
- 2 cups basil leaves
- Juice from 1 lemon, freshly squeezed
- 3 cloves of garlic, minced
- ½ cup cashew nuts, soaked in water overnight then drained
- Salt to taste

Directions:
1. Place a zucchini strips on a plate.
2. Place the rest of the ingredients in a food processor and pulse until smooth.
3. Pour sauce over the zucchini then serve.

Nutrition Information:
Calories per serving: 101; Protein: 3.1g; Carbs: 6.6g; Fat: 7.8g Sugar: 1g

Fueling Recipes

No Bake Optavia Fueling Peanut Butter Brownies

Serves: 6
Cooking Time: 30 minutes

Ingredients:
- 3 tablespoons peanut butter
- 1 cup water
- 6 packets Optavia Double Chocolate Brownie Fueling

Directions:
1. Put all ingredients in a bowl and mix until all ingredients are well incorporated.
2. Pour into silicone molds and place in the freezer.
3. Freeze for 30 minutes before eating.

Nutrition Information:
Calories per serving: 906; Protein: 8.7g; Carbs: 157g; Fat: 31.8g Sugar: 1.5g

Optavia Homemade Bars

Serves: 16
Cooking Time: 2 minutes

Ingredients:
- ½ cup dried blueberries
- ½ cup dried cranberries
- ½ cup unsweetened coconut
- ¼ cup hemp seeds
- ¼ cup chia seeds
- ¼ cup pumpkin seeds
- ½ cup peanut butter, unsweetened
- ¼ cup honey
- 3 packet Medifast Maple and Brown Sugar Oatmeal

Directions:
1. Place all ingredients in a bowl. Mix until everything is well-combined.
2. Place into a dish and press firmly.
3. Put in the fridge to set.
4. Slice into small bars.

Nutrition Information:
Calories per serving:165; Protein:4.5 g; Carbs: 22.3g; Fat: 7.4g Sugar: 10.4g

Greek Yogurt Breakfast Bark

Serves: 2
Cooking Time: 5 minutes

Ingredients:
- 12 ounces plain low-fat Greek yogurt
- 2 packets zero-calorie sugar substitute
- 1 sachet Optavia Essential Red Berry Crunchy O's Cereal

Directions:
1. Line an 8x8 baking dish with non-stick foil. Set aside.
2. In a bowl, combine the Greek yogurt and sugar substitute.
3. Spread the Greek yogurt mixture into the prepared baking dish and sprinkle with the Red Berry Crunchy O's Cereal on top.
4. Put in the freezer for 5 hours until the bark is hard.
5. Break the bark with a sharp knife into smaller pieces.

Nutrition Information:
Calories per serving: 198; Protein: 11.1g; Carbs: 31.2g; Fat: 3.1g Sugar: 15.4g

Silky Peanut Butter Cookies

Serves: 8
Cooking Time: 12 minutes

Ingredients:
- 4 sachets Optavia Essential Silky Peanut Butter Shake
- ¼ teaspoon baking powder
- ¼ cup unsweetened vanilla almond or cashew milk
- 1 tablespoon butter, softened
- ¼ teaspoon vanilla extract
- 1/8 teaspoon sea salt

Directions:
1. Preheat the oven to 350^0F.
2. In a bowl, mix the Essential Silky Peanut Butter Shake and baking powder.
3. Add the milk, butter, and vanilla.
4. Mix until well-combined and a dough is formed.
5. Line a baking sheet with parchment paper.
6. Use a spoon and scoop dough and form small balls.
7. Place the cookie balls on the prepared baking sheet and flatten using a fork.
8. Sprinkle with sea salt on top.
9. Bake for 12 minutes or until the edges are lightly browned.

Nutrition Information:
Calories per serving: 87; Protein: 2.9g; Carbs: 7.2g; Fat: 2.1g Sugar: 1.6g

Greek Yogurt Cookie Dough

Serves: 1
Cooking Time: 5 minutes

Ingredients:
- 1 sachet Optavia Essential Chewy Chocolate Chip Cookie
- 1/2-ounce low fat plain Greek yogurt

Directions:
1. Place all ingredients in a bowl until well combined.
2. Place on a container and chill in the fridge for an hour before serving.

Nutrition Information:
Calories per serving: 81; Protein: 1.4g; Carbs: 11.4g; Fat: 3.4g Sugar: 2.3g

Optavia Biscuit Pizza

Serves: 2
Cooking Time: 15 minutes

Ingredients:
- 1 sachet Optavia Buttermilk Cheddar and Herb Biscuit
- 2 tablespoons water
- 1 tablespoon tomato sauce
- 1 tablespoon low fat cheese, shredded

Directions:
1. Preheat the oven or toaster to 350^0F for 5 minutes.
2. In a bowl, stir the Optavia Buttermilk Cheddar and Herb Biscuit with water to form a thick paste. Spread into a thin circle on a baking tray lined with parchment paper.
3. Cook for 10 minutes to harden.
4. Once harden, spread tomato sauce on top and cheese. Bake for another 5 minutes.

Nutrition Information:
Calories per serving: 437; Protein: 9.5g; Carbs: 68.5g; Fat: 5.3g Sugar: 4.3g

Optavia Granola

Serves: 3
Cooking Time:8 minutes

Ingredients:
- 1 package Medifast or Optavia Oatmeal
- 1 packet stevia
- 1 teaspoon vanilla extract
- ½ teaspoon apple spice or pumpkin pie spice

Directions:
1. Preheat the oven to 400^0F.
2. In a bowl, combine all ingredients and add enough water to get the granola to stick together.
3. Drop the granola onto a cookie sheet lined with parchment paper.
4. Bake for 8 minutes but make sure to give the granola a good shake for even browning halfway through the cooking time.

Nutrition Information:
Calories per serving: 209; Protein: 5.8g; Carbs: 42g; Fat: 3.2g Sugar: 6.2g

Optavia Bread Pudding

Serves: 3
Cooking Time: 30 minutes

Ingredients:
- 1 packet Medifast Maple and Brown Sugar Oatmeal
- 1 packet Medifast Vanilla Pudding
- 1 packet stevia
- ¾ cup water
- ¼ teaspoon baking powder
- ¼ teaspoon vanilla extract
- ¼ teaspoon cinnamon
- ½ cup egg substitute
- 2 tablespoon Walden Farms Caramel Syrup

Directions:
1. Preheat the oven to 350^0F.
2. Mix all ingredients in a bowl until well combined.
3. Pour into a glass dish.
4. Place in the oven and bake for 30 minutes.
5. Remove from the oven and allow to rest before slicing the bread pudding.

Nutrition Information:
Calories per serving: 216; Protein: 7.2g; Carbs: 43.2g; Fat: 2.6g Sugar: 16.3g

Optavia Fueling Mashed Potato Buns

Serves: 3
Cooking Time: 12 minutes

Ingredients:
- 2 egg whites
- 1 Optavia Mashed Potatoes (1 Fueling)
- 1 teaspoon baking powder

Directions:
1. Preheat the oven to 350^0F for five minutes.
2. In a bowl, whisk the egg whites until foamy. Add the Optavia Mashed Potatoes and baking powder. Whisk again until well-combined.
3. Pour into a Ziploc bag and pipe into a bagel mold or donut mold.
4. Place in an oven and bake for 12 minutes.

Nutrition Information:
Calories per serving: 195; Protein: 7.3g; Carbs: 41.9g; Fat: 0.3g Sugar: 2.5g

Optavia Mashed Garlic Potato Pancakes

Serves: 4
Cooking Time: 6 minutes

Ingredients:
- 1 packet Garlic Mashed Potatoes (1 Fueling)
- ¼ teaspoon baking powder
- ¼ cup reduced fat cheese, optional
- ½ cup water

Directions:
1. Combine all ingredients in a bowl until well-combined.
2. Allow the mixture to stand for 5 minutes until it thickens up.
3. Spray the cast iron skillet with cooking spray and heat over medium flame.
4. Spoon mixture into the skillet to form pancakes.
5. Cook for 3 minutes on each side or until lightly golden.

Nutrition Information:
Calories per serving: 310; Protein: 9.8g; Carbs: 64.7g; Fat: 2.1g Sugar: 2.9g

Optavia Fueling Mousse

Serves: 2
Cooking Time: 3 minutes

Ingredients:
- 1 packet Medifast or Optavia hot cocoa
- ½ cup sugar-free gelatin
- 1 tablespoon light cream cheese
- 2 tablespoons cold water
- ¼ cup crushed ice

Directions:
1. Place all ingredients in a blender. Pulse until smooth.
2. Pour into glass and place in the fridge to set.
3. Serve chilled.

Nutrition Information:
Calories per serving: 156; Protein: 5.7g; Carbs: 17.6g; Fat: 3.7g Sugar: 4.5g

Optavia Chocolate Crunch Cookies

Serves: 1
Cooking Time: 2 minutes

Ingredients:
- 1 packet Medifast Brownie Mix
- 3 tablespoons water
- 1 packet peanut butter chocolate crunch bar of your choice

Directions:
1. In a bowl, combine thee Medifast Brownie Mix and water until well combined. Set aside.
2. Place the crunch bar on a heat-proof dish or ramekin and pour over the Brownie Mix.
3. Place in a microwave oven and cook for 2 minutes.

Nutrition Information:
Calories per serving: 997; Protein: 28.9g; Carbs: 125g; Fat: 32g Sugar: 8.3g

Peanut Butter Brownie Ice Cream Sandwiches

Serves: 2
Cooking Time: 2 minutes

Ingredients:
- 1 packet Medifast Brownie Mix
- 3 tablespoons water
- 1 Peanut Butter Crunch Bar or any bar of your choice
- 2 tablespoons Peanut Butter Powder
- 1 tablespoon water
- 2 tablespoons cool whip

Directions:
1. Melt the Brownie Mix with water. Add in the Peanut Butter Crunch until a dough is formed.
2. Spoon 4 dough balls on a plate and flatten using the palm of your hands. Make sure that the dough is ¼ inch thick.
3. Place in a microwave oven and cook for 2 minutes.
4. Meanwhile, mix the Peanut Butter Powder and water to form a paste. Add cool whip. Set aside in the fridge to chill for at least 1 hour.
5. Take the cookies out from the microwave oven and allow to cool.
6. Once cooled, spoon the Peanut Butter ice cream in between two cookies.
7. Serve immediately.

Nutrition Information:
Calories per serving: 410; Protein: 8.3g; Carbs: 57.6g; Fat: 13.2g Sugar: 5.3g

Peanut Butter Crunch Cups

Serves: 4
Cooking Time: 2 minutes

Ingredients:
- 1 packet Optavia Chocolate Pudding
- 3 tablespoons water
- 3 Optavia Peanut Butter Crunch Bars

Directions:
1. Place Optavia Chocolate Pudding and water in a bowl and mix until well combined. Set aside.
2. Place the peanut butter crunch bars in another bowl and microwave for 20 second until melted.
3. Pour the melted peanut butter crunch bars into the pudding mix and whisk until combined.
4. Pour the mixture into silicone muffin cup holders and freeze for 2 hours.

Nutrition Information:
Calories per serving:213; Protein: 2.5g; Carbs: 35.8g; Fat: 6.7g Sugar:3.4 g

Cinnamon Blondies

Serves: 6
Cooking Time: 15 minutes

Ingredients:
- 1 packet Medifast Cinnamon Pretzels
- ¼ teaspoon baking powder
- 1 tablespoon eggbeaters or egg substitute
- 1 tablespoon water
- 1/8 teaspoon cinnamon
- 1 packet stevia

Directions:
1. Preheat the oven to 350°F.
2. While still in the bag, break the pretzels into smaller pieces or place them in a food processor and grind them into powder.
3. Transfer to a bowl and add in the baking powder, eggbeaters, and water. Stir until well combined. Add the rest of the ingredients and mix until a dough is formed.
4. Press the dough into a baking dish.
5. Place in the oven and bake for 15 minutes.
6. Remove from the oven and allow to cool before slicing into bars.

Nutrition Information:
Calories per serving: 264; Protein: 6.7g; Carbs: 54.1g; Fat: 2.4g Sugar: 0.3g

Optavia Haystacks

Serves: 2
Cooking Time: 5 minutes

Ingredients:
- 1 packet Optavia or Medifast Hot Cocoa or Brownie Mix
- 3 tablespoons water
- 1 packet Medifast Cinnamon Pretzel Sticks, crushed
- 2 tablespoons Peanut Butter Powder
- 1 packet Stevia

Directions:
1. In a small bowl, mix together the Medifast Hot Cocoa or Brownie Mix with water to form a paste.
2. Add the rest of the ingredients. Stir until well-combined.
3. Drop a tall pile (about 5 inches) of the mixture into a plate and freeze for at least 30 minutes to an hour or until it hardens.

Nutrition Information:
Calories per serving: 835; Protein: 16.3g; Carbs: 158g; Fat: 12.3g Sugar: 3.5g

Banana Cheesecake Chocolate Cookies

Serves: 2
Cooking Time: 2 minutes

Ingredients:
- 1 packet Optavia Brownie Mix
- 5 tablespoons water
- 1 packet Optavia Banana Pudding Mix
- 2 tablespoons light cream cheese

Directions:
1. Combine the Optavia Brownie Mix and 2 tablespoons of water in a bowl until a thick paste is formed.
2. Spread the mixture into a baking dish or plate until thick round circles are formed.
3. Microwave for 1 minute and 30 seconds until the cookie hardens. Set aside to cool completely.
4. In another bowl, combine the remaining ingredients and mix until a smooth batter is formed.
5. Spread the batter on to the cookies.

Nutrition Information:
Calories per serving: 342; Protein:22.1 g; Carbs: 45.2g; Fat:5.7 g Sugar: 8.2g

Optavia Crunchy Peanut Butter Ice Cream

Serves: 3
Cooking Time: 3 minutes

Ingredients:
- 1 packet Medifast Vanilla Pudding
- ½ cup water
- 2 tablespoons Peanut Butter Powder
- 1 tablespoon light cream cheese
- 1 packet Medifast Pretzels, Crushed

Directions:
1. Mix together the Vanilla Pudding, water, and Peanut Butter Powder until a thick past is formed.
2. Stir in the cream cheese and crushed pretzels.
3. Pour into a container.
4. Freeze for 4 hours or more before serving.

Nutrition Information:
Calories per serving: 300; Protein: 4.3g; Carbs: 60.1g; Fat: 4.8g Sugar: 9.3g

Cheesecake Ice Cream

Serves: 2
Cooking Time: 3 minutes

Ingredients:
- 1 packet Medifast Vanilla Pudding
- ½ cup water
- 1 tablespoon light cream cheese
- ½ teaspoon lemon extract

Directions:
1. Combine all ingredients in a bowl until well-incorporated.
2. Pour into a lidded container and freeze for an hour.
3. Serve cold.

Nutrition Information:
Calories per serving: 189; Protein: 0.7g; Carbs: 41.5g; Fat: 2.3g Sugar: 11.4g

Peanut Butter Brownies and Greek Yogurt Batter

Serves: 2
Cooking Time: 3 minutes

Ingredients:
- 1 packet Medifast Brownie Mix
- 5-ounce low fat plain Greek yogurt
- 1 tablespoon Peanut Butter Powder

Directions:
1. Combine all ingredients in a bowl until well-incorporated.
2. Place mixture in a bowl and chill before serving.

Nutrition Information:
Calories per serving: 597; Protein: 9.2g; Carbs: 100.4g; Fat: 10.3g Sugar: 6.5g

Chocolate Mint Soft Serve Brownie Bottoms

Serves: 2
Cooking Time: 1 minute

Ingredients:
- 1 packet Medifast Brownie Mix
- 1 packet Medifast Chocolate Mint Soft Serve Mix
- ½ cup water

Directions:
1. Place all ingredients in a bowl.
2. Stir until well combined.
3. Place in a microwaveable container and microwave for 50 seconds.
4. Place in container and allow to cool for an hour before serving.

Nutrition Information:
Calories per serving: 585; Protein: 7.1g; Carbs: 103g; Fat: 12.4g Sugar: 7.1g

Chocolate Chip Coffee Cake Muffins

Serves: 4
Cooking Time: 2 minutes

Ingredients:
- 1 packet Medifast Cappuccino
- 1 packet Medifast Chocolate Chip Pancakes
- 1 packet Stevia
- 1 tablespoon eggbeaters
- ¼ teaspoon baking powder
- ¼ cup water

Directions:
1. Mix all ingredients until well-combined.
2. Pour into 4-inch round ramekins.
3. Microwave for 1 minute and 45 seconds.
4. Top with cream cheese if desired.

Nutrition Information:
Calories per serving: 128; Protein: 4.6g; Carbs: 13.8g; Fat: 6.5g Sugar: 4.2g

Optavia Pancake Crepes

Serves: 3
Cooking Time: 6 minutes

Ingredients:
- 1 packet Medifast Chocolate Chip Pancake Mix
- ¼ cup water
- ¼ cup skim ricotta cheese
- ½ packet stevia powder
- 1/8 teaspoon vanilla extract

Directions:
1. Combine the Medifast Chocolate Chip Pancake Mix and water to create a thick paste or batter.
2. Spray a non-stick skillet with cooking spray and pour batter into the pan. Cook for 3 minutes on each side. Set aside.
3. In another bowl, combine the ricotta cheese, stevia powder and vanilla extract.
4. Spread over one side of the pancake and roll to create a crepe.

Nutrition Information:
Calories per serving: 360; Protein: 5.4g; Carbs: 45.1g; Fat: 10.8g Sugar: 0.4g

Optavia Lemon Meringue Bites

Serves: 2
Cooking Time: 2 minutes

Ingredients:
- 2 packets Optavia Essential Lemon Crisp Bars
- 1 ½ cups low fat plain Greek yogurt
- 1 3-ounce box sugar-free lemon gelatin
- ½ teaspoon lime zest

Directions:
1. Line a muffin tin with cupcake liner.
2. Break the Optavia Essential Lemon Crisp Bars into thirds and place in a bowl. Microwave for 15 seconds until soft.
3. Press the softened bars into the cupcake liners to form a crust.
4. In another microwavable-safe bowl, mix the yogurt, gelatin, and lime zest. Microwave for 2 minutes and pour the mixture into the crust-lined cupcake liners.
5. Chill for an hour before serving.

Nutrition Information:
Calories per serving: 326; Protein: 11.9g; Carbs: 45.4g; Fat: 11.2g Sugar: 10.1g

Medifast Fudge Balls

Serves: 4
Cooking Time: 2 minutes

Ingredients:
- 1 packet Medifast Chocolate Shake, divided
- 1 packet Medifast Chocolate Pudding
- 1 tablespoon Walden Farms caramel or chocolate syrup
- 1 tablespoons P2B
- ¼ cup water

Directions:
1. Combine half of the Chocolate Shake, Chocolate Pudding, caramel syrup, and PB2 in a bowl. Add water gradually to form dry dough.
2. Form balls from the mixture using your hands and roll the balls on the remaining chocolate shake powder.
3. Chill before serving.

Nutrition Information:
Calories per serving: 168; Protein: 4.3g; Carbs: 25.2g; Fat: 5.9g Sugar: 7.4g

Chocolate Peanut Butter Cup

Serves: 2
Cooking Time: 3 minutes

Ingredients:
- 2 tablespoons PB2
- 1 packet of Stevia
- Water
- 1 packet Optavia Hot Cocoa or Brownie Mix

Directions:
1. Mix two tablespoons of PB2 and stevia with 1 ½ tablespoons water until creamy. Set aside.
2. In another bowl, mix the Hot Cocoa Powder with 3 tablespoons water. Spread half of the mixture over the bottom of the ramekin.
3. Spread the PB2 over the chocolate bottom layer. Spread the rest of the Cocoa Mixture over the top of the PB2 mixture.
4. Place in the freezer and chill for an hour.

Nutrition Information:
Calories per serving: 778; Protein: 8.9g; Carbs: 126.8g; Fat: 15.3g Sugar: 7.7g

Soft Serve Cookies

Serves: 4
Cooking Time: 12 minutes

Ingredients:
- ½ teaspoon baking powder
- 2 tablespoon eggbeaters
- 3 tablespoons water
- 1 soft serve

Directions:
1. Preheat the oven to 350^0F.
2. Combine all ingredients until well-combined to create a dough.
3. Drop the cookies by spoonful and bake for 12 minutes.
4. Allow to cool.

Nutrition Information:
Calories per serving: 95; Protein: 2.1g; Carbs: 5.8g; Fat: 7.2g Sugar: 3.9g

Maple Rolls

Serves: 3
Cooking Time: 15 minutes

Ingredients:
- 3 packets Medifast Maple and Brown Sugar Oatmeal
- ¾ teaspoon baking powder
- 1 teaspoon maple extract
- 1 packet stevia
- 1 teaspoon vanilla extract
- ¼ cup water

Directions:
1. Mix all ingredients except water in a bowl. Gradually add water until a sticky dough is formed.
2. Divide the dough into three logs.
3. Place in a parchment-lined baking sheet and cook in a 350^{0}F preheated oven for 15 minutes.
4. Allow to cool before serving.

Nutrition Information:
Calories per serving: 170; Protein: 3.9g; Carbs: 35.9g; Fat: 1.7g Sugar: 8.3g

Oatmeal Raisin Cookies

Serves: 4
Cooking Time: 15 minutes

Ingredients:
- 1 packet Medifast Oatmeal
- 1 packet Medifast Oatmeal Raisin Crunch Bar
- 1/8 teaspoon cinnamon
- 1 packet stevia
- 1/3 cup water
- 1/8 teaspoon baking powder
- ½ teaspoon vanilla
- 2 tablespoons PB2

Directions:
1. Preheat the oven to 350^0F.
2. Microwave the Oatmeal Raisin Bar for 15 seconds until melted.
3. Mix the melted bar with the rest of the ingredients until well combined. Let the dough sit for 5 minutes.
4. Line a cookie sheet with parchment paper.
5. Drop dough by spoonful to make 4 cookies.
6. Bake for 15 minutes.

Nutrition Information:
Calories per serving: 137; Protein: 2.5g; Carbs: 20.6g; Fat: 5g Sugar: 2.4g

Cadbury Crème Eggs

Serves: 2
Cooking Time: 5 minutes

Ingredients:
- 1 packet Medifast Hot Cocoa Powder
- 2 tablespoons water
- 1 tablespoon Walden Farms Marshmallow Crème
- 1 tablespoon PB2

Directions:
1. In a bowl, combine the Medifast Hot Cocoa Powder and water. Spoon half of the mixture on a plate and form an oval shape.
2. In another bowl, combine the Marshmallow Crème and PB2. Spoon on top of the oval shaped Cocoa Powder mixture.
3. Pour the remaining half of the chocolate syrup over the top of the Marshmallow Crème mixture.
4. Place in the fridge for at least an hour for the mixture to harden.

Nutrition Information:
Calories per serving: 199; Protein: 5.1g; Carbs: 34g; Fat: 2g Sugar: 13g

CPSIA information can be obtained
at www.ICGtesting.com
Printed in the USA
BVHW012236260322
632563BV00003B/170